Ultimate Dash Diet Plan

Delicious Recipes to Lower Blood Pressure and Improve Your Health

Eleonore Barlow

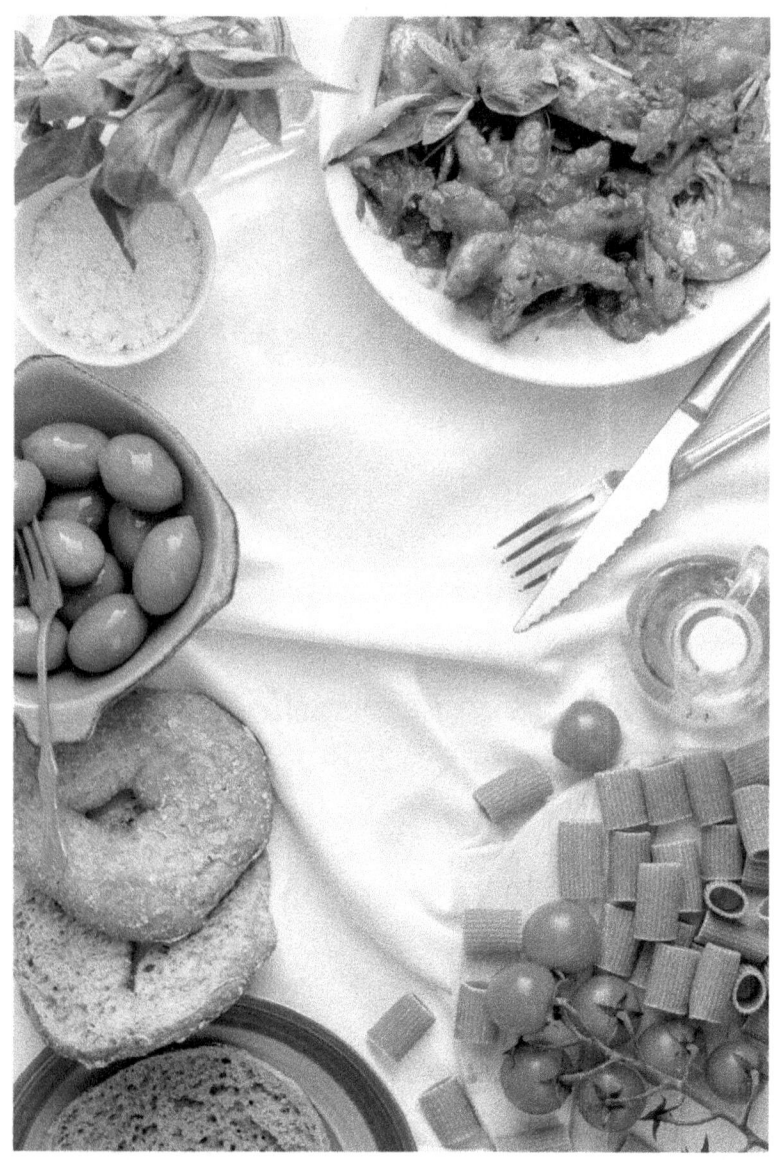

© Copyright 2021 - All rights reserved.

The content contained within this book may not be reproduced, duplicated or transmitted without direct written permission from the author or the publisher.
Under no circumstances will any blame or legal responsibility be held against the publisher, or author, for any damages, reparation, or monetary loss due to the information contained within this book. Either directly or indirectly.

Legal Notice:
This book is copyright protected. This book is only for personal use. You cannot amend, distribute, sell, use, quote or paraphrase any part, or the content within this book, without the consent of the author or publisher.

Disclaimer Notice:
Please note the information contained within this document is for educational and entertainment purposes only. All effort has been executed to present accurate, up to date, and reliable, complete information. No warranties of any kind are declared or implied. Readers acknowledge that the author is not engaging in the rendering of legal, financial, medical or professional advice. The content within this book has been derived from various sources. Please consult a licensed professional before attempting any techniques outlined in this book.
By reading this document, the reader agrees that under no circumstances is the author responsible for any losses, direct or indirect, which are incurred as a result of the use of information contained within this document, including, but not limited to, — errors, omissions, or inaccuracies.

Table of Contents

CARROT AND ZUCCHINI OATMEAL 6

BLUEBERRY AND WALNUT "STEEL" OATMEAL 8

SHRIMP AND EGG MEDLEY 10

CRISPY WALNUT CRUMBLES 12

CHEESY ZUCCHINI OMELETTE 14

OLD FASHIONED BREAKFAST OATMEAL 16

HEALTHY PEACH OATMEAL 18

CRAZY LAMB SALAD 20

HEARTY ROASTED CAULIFLOWER 22

COOL CABBAGE FRIED BEEF 24

FENNEL AND FIGS LAMB 26

BLACK BERRY CHICKEN WINGS 28

MUSHROOM AND OLIVE "MEDITERRANEAN" STEAK 30

ORANGE AND CHILI GARLIC SAUCE 32

TANTALIZING MUSHROOM GRAVY 34

EVERYDAY VEGETABLE STOCK 36

GRILLED CHICKEN WITH LEMON AND FENNEL 38

CARAMELIZED PORK CHOPS AND ONION 41

HEALTHY CAULIFLOWER SALAD 43

CHICKPEA SALAD 45

DASHING BOK CHOY SAMBA 48

SIMPLE AVOCADO CAPRESE SALAD 50

THE RUTABAGA WEDGE DISH 52

RED COLESLAW 54

CLASSIC TUNA SALAD 56

EASY GARLIC ALMOND BUTTER SHRIMP 58

BLACKENED TILAPIA 60

LIGHT LOBSTER BISQUE	62
HERBAL SHRIMP RISOTTO	64
THAI PUMPKIN SEAFOOD STEW	66
PISTACHIO SOLE FISH	68
GARLIC COTTAGE CHEESE CRISPY	70
TASTY CUCUMBER BITES	72
JUICY SIMPLE LEMON FAT BOMBS	74
CHOCOLATE COCONUT BOMBS	76
TERRIFIC JALAPENO BACON BOMBS	78
YUMMY ESPRESSO FAT BOMBS	80
CRISPY COCONUT BOMBS	82
THE SWEET POTATO ACID BUSTER	84
THE SUNSHINE OFFERING	86
THE SLEEPY BUG SMOOTHIE	88
MATCHA COCONUT SMOOTHIE	90
RAVISHING APPLE AND CUCUMBER GLASS	92
CREATIVE WINTER SMOOTHIE	94
THE HEARTY GARLIC AND MUSHROOM CRUNCH	96
EASY PEPPER JACK CAULIFLOWER	98
THE BRUSSELS PLATTER	100
THE CRAZY SOUTHERN SALAD	102
KALE AND CARROT WITH TAHINI DRESSING	104
CRISPY KALE	106

Carrot and Zucchini Oatmeal

Serving: 3

Prep Time: 10 minutes

Cook Time: 8 hours

Ingredients:

½ cup steel cut oats

1 cup coconut milk

1 carrot, grated

¼ zucchini, grated

Pinch of nutmeg

½ teaspoon cinnamon powder

2 tablespoons brown sugar

¼ cup pecans, chopped

How To:

1. Grease the Slow Cooker well.

2.   Add oats, zucchini, milk, carrot, nutmeg, cloves, sugar, cinnamon and stir well.

3.   Place lid and cook on LOW for 8 hours.

4. Divide amongst serving bowls and enjoy!

Nutrition (Per Serving)

Calories: 200

Fat: 4g

Carbohydrates: 11g

Protein: 5g

Blueberry and Walnut "Steel" Oatmeal

Serving: 8

Prep Time: 5 minutes

Cook Time: 7-8 hours

Ingredients:

2 cups steel-cut oats

6 cups water

2 cups low-fat milk

2 cups fresh blueberries

1 ripe banana, mashed

1 teaspoon vanilla extract

2 teaspoons ground cinnamon

2 tablespoons brown sugar

Pinch of salt

½ cup walnuts, chopped

How To:

1. Grease the within of your Slow Cooker.

2. Add oats, milk, water, blueberries, banana, vanilla, sugar, cinnamon and salt to your Slow Cooker.

3. Stir.

4. Place lid and cook on LOW for 7-8 hours.

5. Serve warm with a garnish of chopped walnuts.

6. Enjoy!

Nutrition (Per Serving)

Calories: 372

Fat: 14g

Carbohydrates: 56g

Protein: 8g

Shrimp and Egg Medley

Serving: 4

Prep Time: 15 minutes

Cook Time: nil

Ingredients:

4 hardboiled eggs, peeled and chopped

1-pound cooked shrimp, peeled and de-veined, chopped

1 sprig fresh dill, chopped

¼ cup mayonnaise

1 teaspoon Dijon mustard

4 fresh lettuce leaves

How To:

1. Take an outsized serving bowl and add the listed ingredients (except lettuce.)

2. Stir well.

3. Serve over bet of lettuce leaves.

4. Enjoy!

Nutrition (Per Serving)

Calories: 292

Fat: 17g

Carbohydrates: 1.6g

Protein: 30g

Crispy Walnut Crumbles

Serving: 10

Prep Time: 10 minutes

Cook Time: 8 minutes

Ingredients:

6 ounces kite ricotta/cashew cheese, grated

2 tablespoons walnuts, chopped

1 tablespoon almond butter

½ tablespoon fresh thyme chopped

How To:

1. Preheat your oven to 350 degrees F.
2. Take two large rimmed baking sheets and line with parchment.
3. Add cheese, almond butter to a kitchen appliance and blend.
4. Add walnuts to the combination and pulse.
5. Take a tablespoon and scoop mix onto a baking sheet.

6. Top them with chopped thymes.

7. Bake for 8 minutes, transfer to a cooling rack.

8. Let it cool for half-hour.

9. Serve and enjoy!

Nutrition (Per Serving)

Calories: 80

Fat: 3g

Carbohydrates: 7g

Protein: 7g

Cheesy Zucchini Omelette

Serving: 3

Prep Time: 10 minutes

Cook Time: 20 minutes

Ingredients:

4 large eggs

2-3 medium zucchinis

1-2 garlic cloves, crushed

4 tablespoons grated cheese Season as needed

How To:

1. Take a bowl and add grated zucchinis, confirm to peel them because the skin is bitter.

2. Take a bowl and break within the eggs, crushed garlic and cheese.

3. Pour the mixture during a hot frypan with a touch little bit of oil and place it over medium heat, keep a lid on.

4. Once the egg is cooked nicely, and therefore the bottom is crispy and golden, serve and luxuriate in with a garnish of chopped parsley.

5. Enjoy!

Nutrition (Per Serving)

Calories: 289

Fat: 20g

Carbohydrates: 7g

Protein: 21g

Old Fashioned Breakfast Oatmeal

Serving: 4

Prep Time: 10 minutes

Cook Time: 5 minutes

Ingredients:

2 ½ cups water

1 cup old fashioned oats

1 cup apple, peeled, cored and chopped

3 tablespoons low-fat butter

2 tablespoons palm sugar

½ teaspoon cinnamon powder

How To:

1. Add water, oats, apple, butter, cinnamon, and sugar to a moment pot.

2. Toss well and lock the lid.

3. Cook on high for five minutes.

4. Release the pressure naturally over 10 minutes.

5. Stir oats and divide into bowls.

6. Enjoy!

Nutrition (Per Serving)

Calories: 191

Fat: 2g

Carbohydrates: 9g

Protein: 5g

Healthy Peach Oatmeal

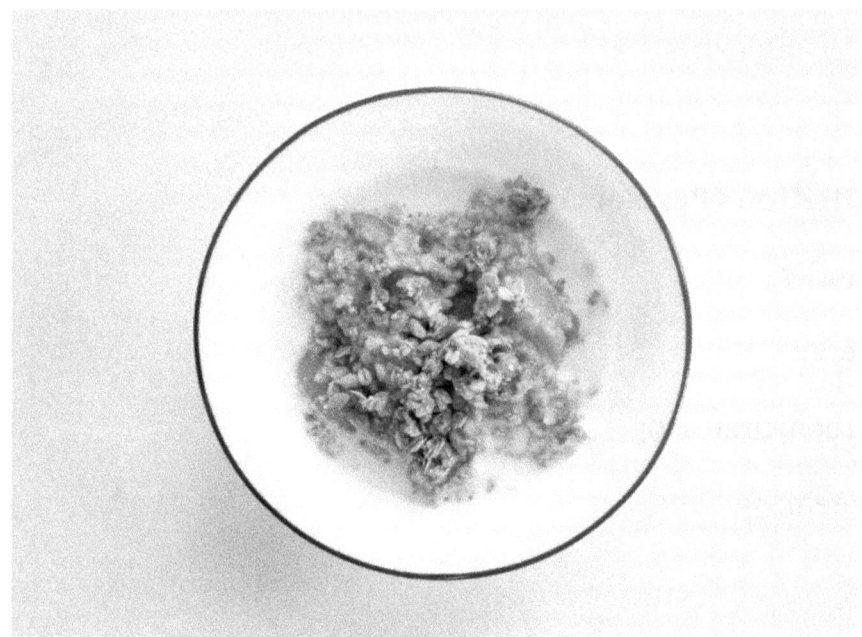

Serving: 8

Prep Time: 10 minutes

Cook Time: 10 minutes

Ingredients:

4 cups old fashioned rolled oats

3 ½ cups low-fat milk

3 ½ cups water

1 teaspoon cinnamon powder

1/3 cup palm sugar

4 peaches, chopped

How To:

1. Add oats, milk, cinnamon, water, sugar, and peaches to your Instant Pot.

2. Toss well.

3. Lock the lid and cook for 10 minutes on high.

4. Release the pressure naturally over 10 minutes.

5. Divide the combination in bowls and serve!

Nutrition (Per Serving)

Calories: 192

Fat: 3g

Carbohydrates: 12g

Protein: 4g

Crazy Lamb Salad

Serving: 4

Prep Time: 10 minutes

Cook Time: 35 minutes

Ingredients:

1 tablespoon olive oil

3-pound leg of lamb, bone removed, leg butterflied Salt and pepper to taste

1 teaspoon cumin

Pinch of dried thyme

2 garlic cloves, peeled and minced For Salad

4 ounces feta cheese, crumbled

½ cup pecans

2 cups spinach

1 ½ tablespoons lemon juice

¼ cup olive oil

1 cup fresh mint, chopped

How To:

1. Rub lamb with salt and pepper, 1 tablespoon oil, thyme, cumin, minced garlic.

2. Pre-heat your grill to medium-high and transfer lamb.

3. Cook for 40 minutes, ensuring to flip it once.

4. Take a lined baking sheet and spread the pecans.

5. Toast in oven for 10 minutes at 350 degree F.

6. Transfer grilled lamb to chopping board and let it cool.

7. Slice.

8. Take a salad bowl and add spinach, 1 cup mint, feta cheese, ¼ cup vegetable oil , juice , toasted pecans, salt, pepper and toss well.

9. Add lamb slices on top.

10. Serve and enjoy!

Nutrition (Per Serving)

Calories: 334

Fat: 33g

Carbohydrates: 5g

Protein: 7g

Hearty Roasted Cauliflower

Serving: 8

Prep Time: 5 minutes

Cook Time: 30 minutes

Ingredients:

1 large cauliflower head

2 tablespoons melted coconut oil

2 tablespoons fresh thyme

1 teaspoon Celtic sea sunflower seeds

1 teaspoon fresh ground pepper

1 head roasted garlic

2 tablespoons fresh thyme for garnish

How To:

1. Pre-heat your oven to 425 degrees F.
2. Rinse cauliflower and trim, core and sliced.
3. Lay cauliflower evenly on rimmed baking tray.

4. Drizzle copra oil evenly over cauliflower, sprinkle thyme leaves.

5. Season with pinch of sunflower seeds and pepper.

6. Squeeze roasted garlic.

7. Roast cauliflower until slightly caramelized for about half-hour, ensuring to show once.

8. Garnish with fresh thyme leaves.

9. Enjoy!

Nutrition (Per Serving)

Calories: 129

Fat: 11g

Carbohydrates: 6g

Protein: 7g

Cool Cabbage Fried Beef

Serving: 4

Prep Time: 5 minutes

Cook Time: 15 minutes

Ingredients:

1-pound beef, ground and lean

½ pound bacon

1 onion

1 garlic clove, minced

½ head cabbage

pepper to taste

How To:

1. Take skillet and place it over medium heat.
2. Add chopped bacon, beef and onion until slightly browned.
3. Transfer to a bowl and keep it covered.

4. Add minced garlic and cabbage to the skillet and cook until slightly browned.

5. Return the bottom beef mix to the skillet and simmer for 3-5 minutes over low heat.

6. Serve and enjoy!

Nutrition (Per Serving)

Calories: 360

Fat: 22g

Net Carbohydrates: 5g

Protein: 34g

Fennel and Figs Lamb

Serving: 2

Prep Time: 10 minutes

Cook Time: 40 minutes

Ingredients:

6 ounces lamb racks 1 fennel bulbs, sliced pepper to taste

1 tablespoon olive oil

2 figs, cut in half

1/8 cup apple cider vinegar

1/2 tablespoon swerve

How To:

1. Take a bowl and add fennel, figs, vinegar, swerve, oil and toss.
2. Transfer to baking dish.
3. Season with sunflower seeds and pepper.
4. Bake for quarter-hour at 400 degrees F.

5. Season lamb with sunflower seeds and pepper and transfer to a heated pan over medium-high heat.

6. Cook for a couple of minutes.

7. Add lamb to the baking dish with fennel and bake for 20 minutes.

8. Divide between plates and serve.

9. Enjoy!

Nutrition (Per Serving)

Calories: 230

Fat: 3g

Carbohydrates: 5g

Protein: 10g

Black Berry Chicken Wings

Serving: 4

Prep Time: 35 minutes

Cook Time: 50minutes

Ingredients:

3 pounds chicken wings, about 20 pieces ½ cup blackberry chipotle jam Pepper to taste

½ cup water

How To:

1. Add water and jam to a bowl and blend well.

2. Place chicken wings during a zip bag and add two-thirds of marinade.

3. Season with pepper.

4. Let it marinate for half-hour.

5. Pre-heat your oven to 400 degrees F.

6. Prepare a baking sheet and wire rack, place chicken wings in wire rack and bake for quarter-hour.

7. Brush remaining marinade and bake for half-hour more.

8. Enjoy!

Nutrition (Per Serving)

Calories: 502

Fat: 39g

Carbohydrates: 01.8g

Protein: 34g

Mushroom and Olive "Mediterranean" Steak

Serving: 2

Prep Time: 10 minutes

Cook Time: 14 minutes

Ingredients:

1/2-pound boneless beef sirloin steak, ¾ inch thick, cut into 4 pieces

1/2 large red onion, chopped

1/2 cup mushrooms

2 garlic cloves, thinly sliced

2 tablespoons olive oil

1/4 cup green olives, coarsely chopped

1/2 cup parsley leaves, finely cut

How To:

Take an outsized sized skillet and place it over medium-high heat.

1. Add oil and let it heat up.

2. Add beef and cook until each side are browned, remove beef and drain fat.

3. Add the remainder of the oil to the skillet and warmth.

4. Add onions, garlic and cook for 2-3 minutes.

5. Stir well.

6. Add mushrooms, olives and cook until the mushrooms are thoroughly done.

7. Return the meat to the skillet and reduce heat to medium.

8. Cook for 3-4 minutes (covered).

9. Stir in parsley.

10. Serve and enjoy!

Nutrition (Per Serving)

Calories: 386

Fat: 30g

Carbohydrates: 11g

Protein: 21g

Orange and Chili Garlic Sauce

Serving: 5 cups

Prep Time: 15 minutes

Cook Time: 8 hours

Ingredients:

½ cup apple cider vinegar

4 pounds red jalapeno peppers, stems, seeds and ribs removed, chopped

10 garlic cloves, chopped

½ cup tomato paste

Juice of 1 orange zest

½ cup honey

2 tablespoons soy sauce

2 teaspoons salt

How To:

1. Add vinegar, garlic, peppers, ingredient , fruit juice , honey, zest, soy and salt to your Slow Cooker.

2. Stir and shut lid.
3. Cook on LOW for 8 hours.
4. Use as required!

Nutrition (Per Serving)

Calories: 33

Fat: 1g

Carbohydrates: 8g

Protein: 1g

Tantalizing Mushroom Gravy

Serving: 2 cups

Prep Time: 5 minutes

Cook Time: 5-8 hours

Ingredients:

1 cup button mushrooms, sliced

¾ cup low-fat buttermilk

1/3 cup water

1 medium onion, finely diced

2 garlic cloves, minced

2 tablespoons extra virgin olive oil

2 tablespoons all-purpose flour

1 tablespoon fresh rosemary, minced Freshly ground black pepper

How To:

1. Add the listed ingredients to your Slow Cooker.

2. Place lid and cook on LOW for 5-8 hours.

3. Serve warm and use as needed!

Nutrition (Per Serving)

Calories: 54

Fat: 4g

Carbohydrates: 4g

Protein: 2g

Everyday Vegetable Stock

Serving: 10 cups

Prep Time: 5 minutes

Cook Time: 8-12 hours

Ingredients:

2 celery stalks (with leaves), quartered

4 ounces mushrooms, with stems

2 carrots, unpeeled and quartered

1 onion, unpeeled, quartered from pole to pole

1 garlic head, unpeeled, halved across middle

2 fresh thyme sprigs

10 peppercorns

½ teaspoon salt

Enough water to fill 3 quarters of Slow Cooker

How To:

1. Add celery, mushrooms, onion, carrots, garlic, thyme, salt, peppercorn and water to your Slow Cooker.

2. Stir and canopy.

3. Cook on LOW for 8-12 hours.

4. Strain the stock through a fine mesh cloth/metal mesh and discard solids.

5. Use as needed.

Nutrition (Per Serving)

Calories: 38

Fat: 5g

Carbohydrates: 1g

Protein: 0g

Grilled Chicken with Lemon and Fennel

Serving: 4

Prep Time: 5 minutes

Cook Time: 25 minutes

Ingredients:

2 cups chicken fillets, cut and skewed

1 large fennel bulb

2 garlic cloves

1 jar green olives

1 lemon

How To:

1. Pre-heat your grill to medium-high.
2. Crush garlic cloves.
3. Take a bowl and add vegetable oil and season with sunflower seeds and pepper.
4. Coat chicken skewers with the marinade.

5. Transfer them under the grill and grill for 20 minutes, ensuring to show them halfway through until golden.

6. Zest half the lemon and cut the opposite half into quarters.

7. Cut the fennel bulb into similarly sized segments.

8. Brush vegetable oil everywhere the clove segments and cook for 3-5 minutes.

9. Chop them and add them to the bowl with the marinade.

10. Add lemon peel and olives.

11. Once the meat is prepared, serve with the vegetable mix.

12. Enjoy!

Nutrition (Per Serving)

Calories: 649

Fat: 16g

Carbohydrates: 33g

Protein: 18g

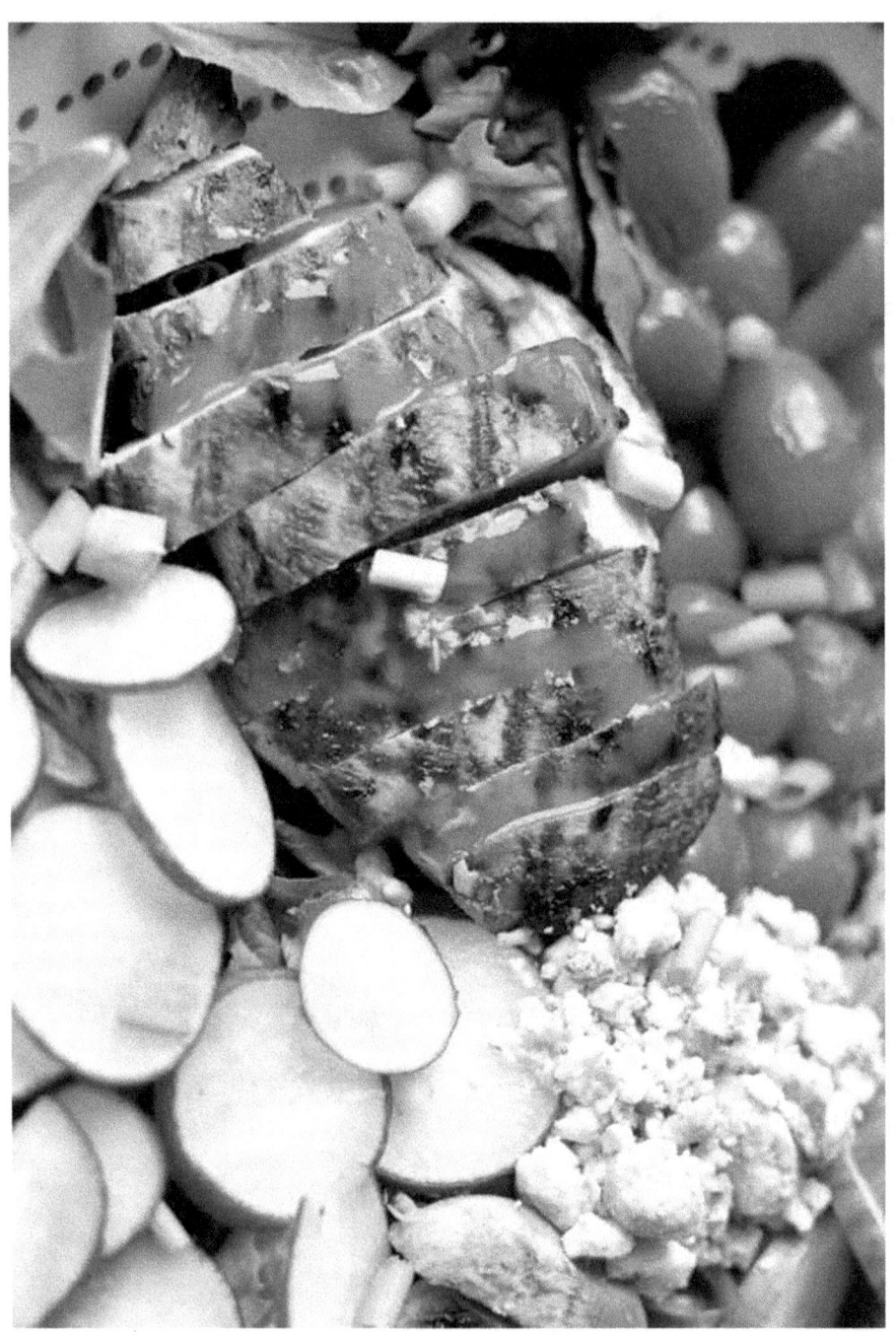

Caramelized Pork Chops and Onion

Serving: 4

Prep Time: 5 minutes

Cook Time: 40 minutes

Ingredients:

4-pound chuck roast

4 ounces green Chili, chopped

2 tablespoons of chili powder

½ teaspoon of dried oregano

½ teaspoon of cumin, ground

2 garlic cloves, minced

How To:

1. Rub the chops with a seasoning of 1 teaspoon of pepper and a couple of teaspoons of sunflower seeds.

2. Take a skillet and place it over medium heat, add oil and permit the oil to heat up.

3. Brown the seasoned chop each side.

4. Add water and onion to the skillet and canopy, lower the warmth to low and simmer for 20 minutes.

5. Turn the chops over and season with more sunflower seeds and pepper.

6. Cover and cook until the water fully evaporates and therefore the beer [MOU1] shows a rather brown texture.

7. Remove the chops and serve with a topping of the caramelized onion.

8. Serve and enjoy!

Nutrition (Per Serving)

Calorie: 47

Fat: 4g

Carbohydrates: 4g

Protein: 0.5g

Healthy Cauliflower Salad

Serving: 4

Prep Time: 10 minutes

Cook Time: nil

Ingredients:

1 head cauliflower, broken into florets

1 small onion, chopped

1/8 cup extra virgin olive oil

¼ cup apple cider vinegar

½ teaspoon sea salt

½ teaspoon black pepper

¼ cup dried cranberries

¼ cup pumpkin seeds

How To:

1. Wash the cauliflower thoroughly and break down into florets.

2. Transfer the florets to a bowl.

3. Take another bowl and whisk in oil, salt, pepper and vinegar.

4. Add pumpkin seeds, cranberries to the bowl with dressing.

5. Mix well and pour dressing over cauliflower florets.

6. Toss well.

7. Add onions and toss.

8. Chill and serve.

9. Enjoy!

Nutrition (Per Serving)

Calories: 163

Fat: 11g

Carbohydrates: 16g

Protein: 3g

Chickpea Salad

Serving: 4

Prep Time: 6 minutes

Cook Time: Nil

Ingredients:

1 cup canned chickpeas, drained and rinsed.

2 spring onions, thinly sliced.

1 small cucumber, diced.

2 green bell peppers, chopped.

2 tomatoes, diced.

2 tablespoons fresh parsley, chopped.

1 teaspoon capers, drained and rinsed.

Half a lemon, juiced.

2 tablespoons sunflower oil.

1 tablespoon red wine vinegar.

Pinch of dried oregano.

Sunflower seeds and pepper to taste

How To:

1.   Take a medium sized bowl and add chickpeas, spring onions, cucumber, bell pepper, tomato, parsley and capers.

2.   Take another bowl and mix in the rest of the ingredients, pour mixture over chickpea salad and toss well.

3.   Coat and serve, enjoy!

Nutrition (Per Serving)

Calories: 74

Fat: 0.7g

Carbohydrates: 16g

Protein: 2g

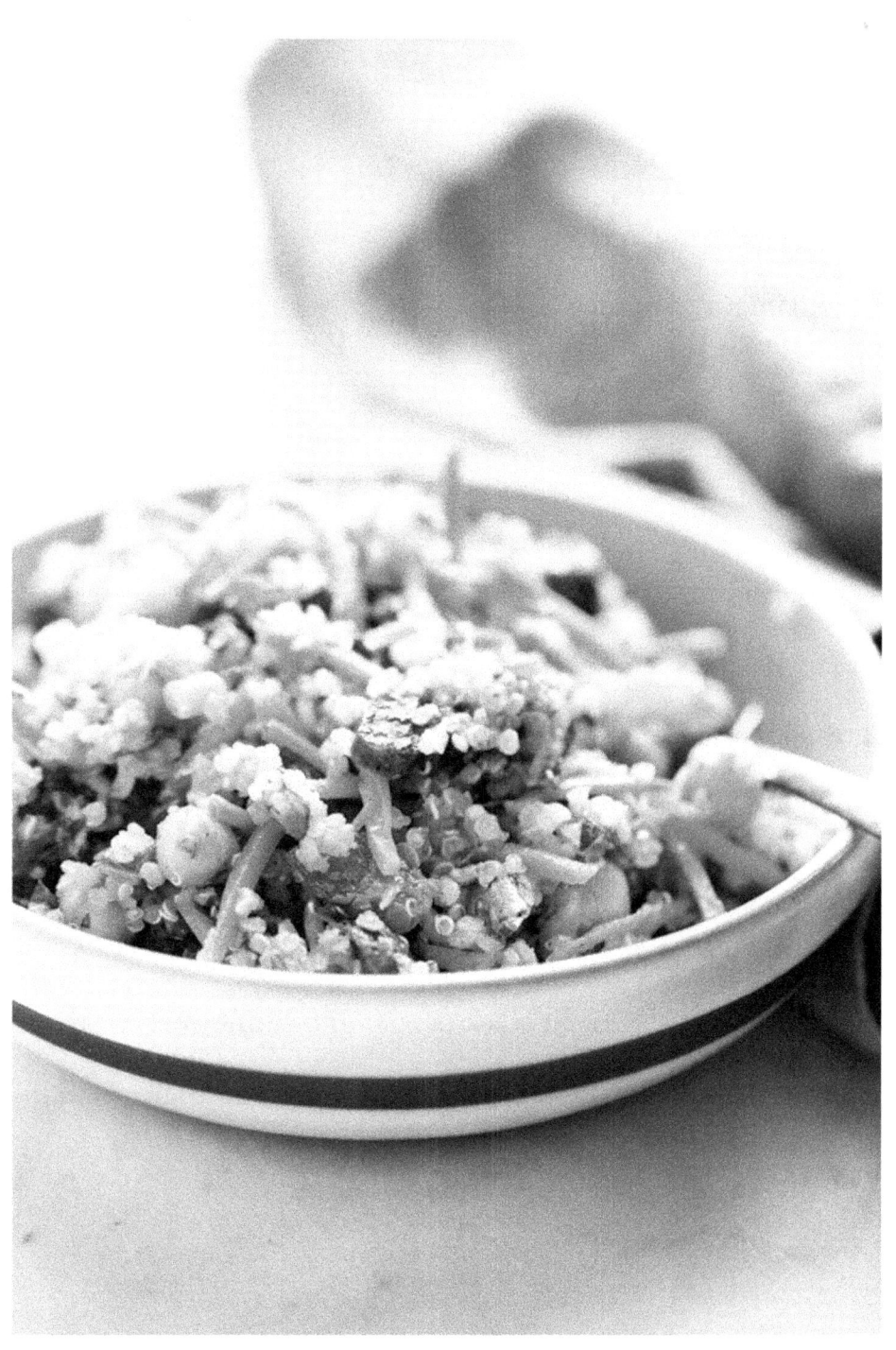

Dashing Bok Choy Samba

Serving: 3

Prep Time: 5 minutes

Cook Time: 15 minutes

Ingredients:

4 bok choy, sliced

1 onion, sliced

½ cup Parmesan cheese, grated

4 teaspoons coconut cream

Sunflower seeds and freshly ground black pepper, to taste

How To:

1. Mix bok choy with black pepper and sunflower seeds.

2. Take a cooking pan, heat the oil and to sauté sliced onion for 5 minutes.

3. Then add cream and seasoned bok choy.

4. Cook for 6 minutes.

5. Stir in Parmesan cheese and cover with a lid.

6. Reduce the heat to low and cook for 3 minutes.

7. Serve warm and enjoy!

Nutrition (Per Serving)

Calories: 112

Fat: 4.9g

Carbohydrates: 1.9g

Protein: 3g

Simple Avocado Caprese Salad

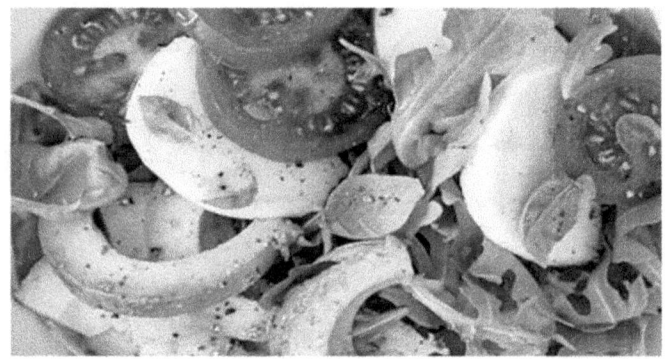

Serving: 6

Prep Time: 15 minutes

Cook Time: 29 minutes

Ingredients:

2 avocados, cubed

1 cup cherry tomatoes, halved

8 ounces mozzarella balls, halved

2 tablespoons finely chopped fresh basil

2 tablespoons olive oil

2 tablespoons balsamic vinegar

1 tablespoon sunflower seeds Fresh ground black pepper

How To:

1. Take a bowl and add the listed ingredients, toss them well until thoroughly mixed.

2. Season with pepper according to your taste.

3. Serve and enjoy!

Nutrition (Per Serving)

Calories: 358

Fat: 30g

Carbohydrates: 9g

Protein: 14g

The Rutabaga Wedge Dish

Serving: 4

Prep Time: 15 minutes

Cook Time: 45 minutes

Ingredients:

2 medium rutabagas, medium, cleaned and peeled

4 tablespoons almond butter

½ teaspoon sunflower seeds

½ teaspoon onion powder

1/8 teaspoon black pepper

½ cup buffalo wing sauce

¼ cup blue cheese dressing, low fat and low sodium 2 green onions, chopped

How To:

1. Pre-heat your oven to 400 degrees F.
2. Line a baking sheet with parchment paper.

3. Wash and peel rutabagas, clean and peel them, and cut into wedge shapes.

4. Take a skillet and place it over low heat, add almond butter and melt.

5. Stir in onion powder, sunflower seeds, onion, black pepper.

6. Use seasoned almond butter to coat wedges.

7. Arrange wedges in a single layer on the baking sheet.

8. Bake for 30 minutes.

9. Remove and coat in buffalo sauce and return to oven.

10. Bake for 15 minutes more.

11. Place wedges on serving plate and trickle with blue cheese dressing.

12. Garnish with chopped green onion and enjoy!

Nutrition (Per Serving)

Calories: 235

Fat: 15g

Carbohydrates: 10g

Protein: 2.5g

Red Coleslaw

Serving: 4

Prep Time: 10 minutes

Cook Time: 0 minutes

Ingredients:

1 2/3 pounds red cabbage

2 tablespoons ground caraway seeds

1 tablespoon whole grain mustard

1 1/4 cups mayonnaise

Sunflower seeds and black pepper

How To:

1. Take a large bowl and all the remaining ingredients.
2. Mix it well and let it sit for 10 minutes.
3. Serve and enjoy!

Nutrition (Per Serving)

Calories: 406

Fat: 40.8g

Carbohydrates: 10g

Protein: 2.2g

Classic Tuna Salad

Serving: 4

Prep Time: 10 minutes

Cook Time: Nil

Ingredients:

12 ounces white tuna, in water

½ cup celery, diced

2 tablespoons fresh parsley, chopped

2 tablespoons low-calorie mayonnaise, low fat and low sodium

½ teaspoon Dijon mustard

½ teaspoon sunflower seeds

¼ teaspoon fresh ground black pepper

Direction

1. Take a medium sized bowl and add tuna, parsley, and celery.

2. Mix well and add mayonnaise and mustard.

3. Season with pepper and sunflower seeds.

4. Stir and add olives, relish, chopped pickle, onion and mix well.

5. Serve and enjoy

Nutrition (Per Serving)

Calories: 137

Fat: 5g

Carbohydrates: 1g

Protein: 20g

Easy Garlic Almond Butter Shrimp

Serving: 4

Prep Time: 15 minutes

Cook Time: 30 minutes

Ingredients:

pounds shrimp

1-2 tablespoons garlic, minced

½ cup almond butter

1 tablespoon lemon pepper seasoning

½ teaspoon garlic powder

How To:

1. Pre-heat your oven to 300 degrees F.
2. Take a bowl and mix in garlic and almond butter.
3. Place shrimp in a pan and dot with almond butter garlic mix.
4. Sprinkle garlic powder and lemon pepper.

5. Bake for 30 minutes.

6. Enjoy!

Nutrition (Per Serving)

Calories: 749

Fat: 30g

Net Carbohydrates: 7g

Protein: 74g

Blackened Tilapia

Serving: 2

Prep Time: 9 minutes

Cook Time: 9 minutes

Ingredients:

1 cup cauliflower, chopped

1 teaspoon red pepper flakes

1 tablespoon Italian seasoning

1 tablespoon garlic, minced

ounces tilapia

cup English cucumber, chopped with peel

tablespoons olive oil

1 sprig dill, chopped

1 teaspoon stevia

tablespoons lime juice

2 tablespoons Cajun blackened seasoning

How To:

1. Take a bowl and add the seasoning ingredients (except Cajun).

2. Add a tablespoon of oil and whip.

3. Pour dressing over cauliflower and cucumber.

4. Brush the fish with olive oil on both sides.

5. Take a skillet and grease it well with 1 tablespoon of olive oil.

6. Press Cajun seasoning on both sides of fish.

7. Cook fish for 3 minutes per side.

8. Serve with vegetables and enjoy!

Nutrition (Per Serving)

Calories: 530

Fat: 33g

Net Carbohydrates: 4g

Protein: 32g

Light Lobster Bisque

Serving: 4

Prep Time: 10 minutes 400

Cook Time: 6 minutes

Ingredients:

1 cup diced carrots

1 cup diced celery

29 ounces diced tomatoes

2 minced whole shallots 1 clove of minced garlic

1 tablespoon butter

32-ounce chicken broth, low-sodium

1 teaspoon dill, dried

1 teaspoon freshly ground black pepper

½ teaspoon paprika

lobster tails

1-pint heavy whipping cream

How To:

1. Add butter, garlic and minced shallots to a microwave safe bowl.

2. Microwave for 2-3 minutes on HIGH.

3. Add tomatoes, celery, carrot, minced shallots, garlic to your Instant Pot.

4. Add chicken broth and spices to the Pot.

5. Use a knife to cut the lobster tails if you prefer and add them to the Instant Pot.

6. Lock the lid and cook on HIGH pressure for 4 minutes.

7. Release the pressure naturally over 10 minutes.

8. Use an immersion blender to puree to your desired chunkiness.

9. Serve and enjoy!

Nutrition (Per Serving)

Calories: 437

Fats: 17g

Carbs: 21g

Protein: 38g

Herbal Shrimp Risotto

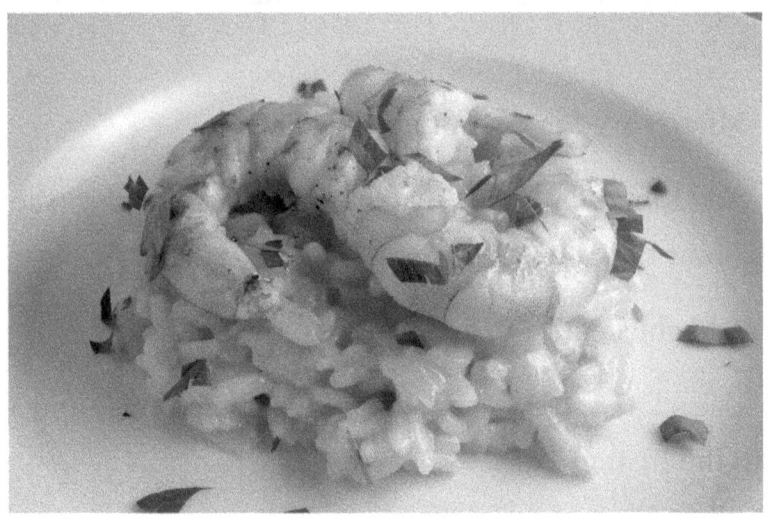

Serving: 4

Prep Time: 10 minutes

Cook Time: 8 minutes

Ingredients:

2 pounds shrimp with their tails removed

cup instant rice

cups vegetable broth

1 chopped up onion

1 cup chicken breast cut into fine strips ¼ cup lemon juice

1 teaspoon crushed red pepper

¼ cup parsley

¼ cup fresh dill

pieces chopped up garlic cloves

1 tablespoon black pepper

½ cup parmesan

1 cup mozzarella cheese

How To:

1. Add the listed ingredients to your Instant Pot and stir.
2. Lock the lid and cook on HIGH pressure for 8 minutes.
3. Release the pressure naturally over 10 minutes.
4. Open lid and top with cheese.
5. Serve hot and enjoy!

Nutrition (Per Serving)

Calories: 463

Fat: 8g

Carbohydrates: 63g

Protein: 29g

Thai Pumpkin Seafood Stew

Serving: 4

Prep Time: 5 minutes

Cook Time: 35 minutes

Ingredients:

1 ½ tablespoons fresh galangal, chopped

1 teaspoon lime zest

1 small kabocha squash

32 medium sized mussels, fresh

1 pound shrimp

16 thai leaves

1 can coconut milk

1 tablespoon lemongrass, minced

garlic cloves, roughly chopped

32 medium clams, fresh

½ pounds fresh salmon

tablespoons coconut oil

Pepper to taste

How To:

1. Add coconut milk, lemongrass, galangal, garlic, lime leaves in a small-sized saucepan, bring to a boil.

2. Let it simmer for 25 minutes.

3. Strain mixture through a fine sieve into the large soup pot and bring to a simmer.

4. Add oil to a pan and heat up, add Kabocha squash.

5. Season with salt and pepper, sauté for 5 minutes.

6. Add mix to coconut mix.

7. Heat oil in a pan and add fish shrimp, season with salt and pepper, cook for 4 minutes.

8. Add mixture to coconut milk, mix alongside clams and mussels.

9. Simmer for 8 minutes, garnish with basil and enjoy!

Nutrition (Per Serving)

Calories: 370

Fat: 16g

Net Carbohydrates: 10g

Protein: 16g

Pistachio Sole Fish

Serving: 4

Prep Time: 5 minutes

Cook Time: 10 minutes

Ingredients:

(5 ounces) boneless sole fillets

Sunflower seeds and pepper as needed

½ cup pistachios, finely chopped

Juice of 1 lemon

1 teaspoon extra virgin olive oil

How To:

1. Pre-heat your oven to 350 degrees F.
2. Line a baking sheet with parchment paper and keep it on the side.
3. Pat fish dry with kitchen towels and lightly season with sunflower seeds and pepper.
4. Take a small bowl and stir in pistachios.

5. Place sole on the prepared baking sheet and press 2 tablespoons of pistachio mixture on top of each fillet.

6. Drizzle fish with lemon juice and olive oil.

7. Bake for 10 minutes until the top is golden and fish flakes with a fork.

8. Serve and enjoy!

Nutrition (Per Serving)

Calories: 166

Fat: 6g

Carbohydrates: 2g

Protein: 26g

Garlic Cottage Cheese Crispy

Serving: 4

Prep Time: 5 minutes

Cook Time: 2 minutes

Ingredients:

1 cup cottage cheese

½ teaspoon Garlic powder

Pinch of pepper

Pinch of onion powder

How To:

1. Take a skillet and place it over medium heat.
2. Take a bowl and mix in cheese and spices.
3. Scoop half a teaspoon of the cheese mix and place in the pan.
4. Cook for 1 minute per side.
5. Repeat until done.

6. Enjoy!

Nutrition (Per Serving)

Calories: 70

Fat: 6g

Carbohydrates: 1g

Protein: 6g

Tasty Cucumber Bites

Serving: 4

Prep Time: 5 minutes

Cook Time: nil

Ingredients:

1 (8 ounce) cream cheese container, low fat

1 tablespoon bell pepper, diced

1 tablespoon shallots, diced

1 tablespoon parsley, chopped

2 cucumbers

Pepper to taste

How To:

1. Take a bowl and add cream cheese, onion, pepper, parsley.

2. Peel cucumbers and cut in half.

3. Remove seeds and stuff with cheese mix.

4. Cut into bite sized portions and enjoy!

Nutrition (Per Serving)

Calories: 85

Fat: 4g

Carbohydrates: 2g

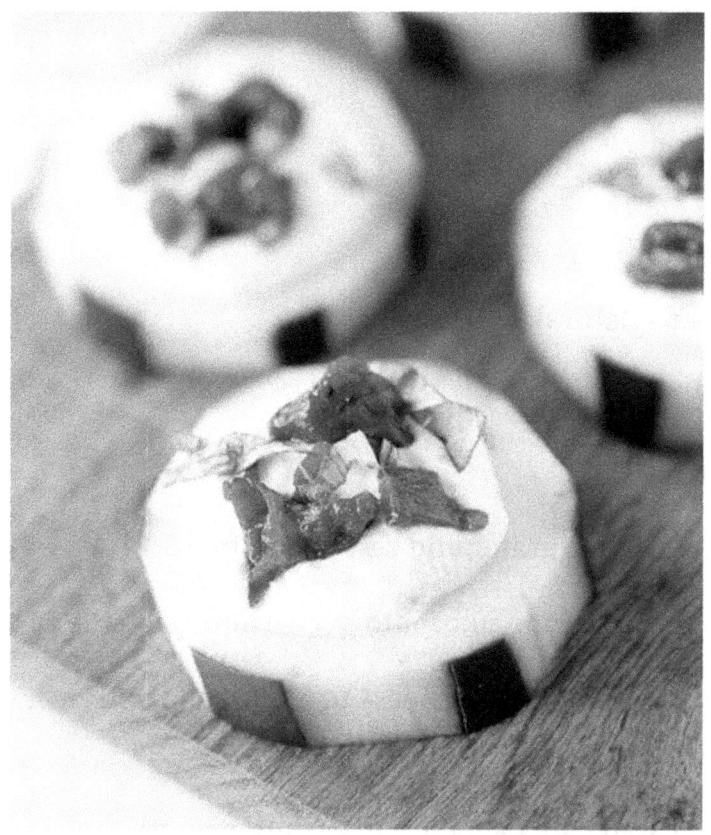

Protein: 3g

Juicy Simple Lemon Fat Bombs

Serving: 3

Prep Time: 10 minutes

Cooking Time: / Freeze Time: 2 hours

Ingredients:

1 whole lemon

4 ounces cream cheese

2 ounces butter

2 teaspoons natural sweetener

How To:

1. Take a fine grater and zest your lemon.

2. Squeeze lemon juice into a bowl alongside the zest.

3. Add butter, cream cheese to a bowl and add zest, salt, sweetener and juice.

4. Stir well using a hand mixer until smooth.

5. Spoon mix into molds and freeze for 2 hours.

6. Serve and enjoy!

Nutrition (Per Serving)

Total Carbs: 4g

Fiber: 1g

Protein: 4g

Fat: 43g

Calories: 404

Chocolate Coconut Bombs

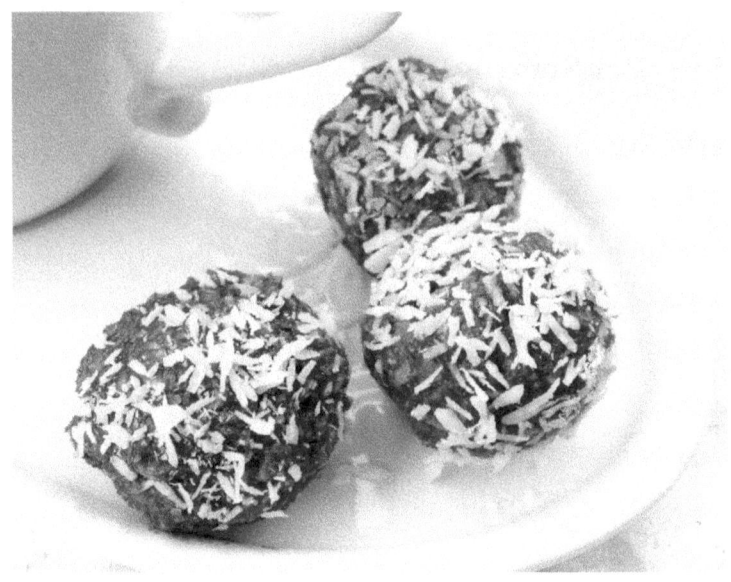

Serving: 12

Prep Time: 20 minutes

Cooking Time: None

Freeze Time: 1 hour

Ingredients:

½ cup dark cocoa powder

½ tablespoon vanilla extract

5 drops stevia

1 cup coconut oil, solid

tablespoon peppermint extract

How To:

1. Take a high-speed food processor and add all the ingredients.

2. Blend until combined.

3. Take a teaspoon and drop a spoonful onto parchment paper.

4. Refrigerate until solidified and keep refrigerated.

Nutrition (Per Serving)

Total Carbs: 0g

Fiber: 0g

Protein: 0g

Fat: 14g

Calories: 126

Terrific Jalapeno Bacon Bombs

Serving: 2

Prep Time: 15 minutes

Cook Time: 10 minutes

Ingredients:

12 large jalapeno peppers

16 bacon strips

6 ounces full fat cream cheese

2 teaspoon garlic powder

1 teaspoon chili powder

How To:

1. Pre-heat your oven to 350 degrees F.

2. Place a wire rack over a roasting pan and keep it on the side.

3. Make a slit lengthways across jalapeno pepper and scrape out the seeds, discard them.

4. Place a nonstick skillet over high heat and add half of your bacon strips, cook until crispy.

5. Drain them.

6. Chop the cooked bacon strips and transfer to large bowl.

7. Add cream cheese and mix.

8. Season the cream cheese and bacon mix with garlic and chili powder.

9. Mix well.

10. Stuff the mix into the jalapeno peppers with and wrap a raw bacon strip all around.

11. Arrange the stuffed wrapped jalapeno on prepared wire rack.

12. Roast for 10 minutes.

13. Transfer to cooling rack and serve!

Nutrition (Per Serving)

Calories: 209

Fat: 9g

Net Carbohydrates: 15g

Protein: 9g

Yummy Espresso Fat Bombs

Serving: 24

Prep Time: 20 minutes

Cooking Time: nil Freeze Time: 4 hours

Ingredients:

5 tablespoons butter, tender

3 ounces cream cheese, soft

2 ounces espresso

4 tablespoons coconut oil

2 tablespoons coconut whipping cream

2 tablespoons stevia

How To:

1. Prepare your double boiler and melt all ingredients (except stevia) for 3-4 minutes and mix.

2. Add sweetener and mix using hand mixer.

3. Spoon mixture into silicone muffin molds and freeze for 4 hours.

4. Remove fat bombs and enjoy!

Nutrition (Per Serving)

Total Carbs: 1.3g

Fiber: 0.2g

Protein: 0.3g

Fat: 7g

Crispy Coconut Bombs

Serving: 6

Prep Time: 10 minutes

Cooking Time: / Freeze Time: 1-2 hours

Ingredients:

14 ½ ounces coconut milk

¾ cup coconut oil

1 cup unsweetened coconut flakes

20 drops stevia

How To:

1. Microwave your coconut oil for 20 seconds in microwave.
2. Mix in coconut milk and stevia in the hot oil.
3. Stir in coconut flakes and pour the mixture into molds.
4. Let it chill for 60 minutes in fridge.
5. Serve and enjoy!

Nutrition (Per Serving)

Total Carbs: 2g

Fiber: 0.5g

Protein: 1g

Fat: 13g

Calories: 123

Net Carbs: 1g

The Sweet Potato Acid Buster

Serving: 2

Prep Time: 5 minutes

Ingredients:

1 cup sweet potato, chopped

1 cup almond milk

¼ teaspoon nutmeg

¼ teaspoon ground cinnamon

1 teaspoon flaxseed

1 small avocado, cubed

Few spinach leaves, torn

Toppings:

Handful of crushed almonds

Handful of crushed cashews

3 tablespoons orange juice

How To:

1. Blend all the ingredients until smooth.

2. Add a few ice cubes to make it chilled.

3. Add your desired toppings.

4. Enjoy!

Nutrition (Per Serving)

Calories: 200

Fat: 10g

Carbohydrates: 14g

Protein 2g

The Sunshine Offering

Serving: 2

Prep Time: 5 minutes

Ingredients:

2 cups fresh spinach

1 ½ cups almond milk ½ cup coconut water

3 cups fresh pineapple

2 tablespoons coconut unsweetened flakes

How To:

1. Add all the listed ingredients to your blender.
2. Blend until smooth.
3. Add a few ice cubes and serve the smoothie.
4. Enjoy!

Nutrition (Per Serving)

Calories: 200

Fat: 10g

Carbohydrates: 14g

Protein 2g

The Sleepy Bug Smoothie

Serving: 2

Prep Time: 5 minutes

Ingredients:

1 cup fennel tea infusion

1 cup almond milk

1 cup watermelon, chopped

1 green apple

½ cup pomegranate

½ inch ginger

Stevia to sweeten

How To:

1. Add the listed ingredients to your blender.
2. Blend until smooth.
3. Add a bit of stevia if you want more sweetness.
4. Serve chilled and enjoy!

Nutrition (Per Serving)

Calories: 200

Fat: 10g

Carbohydrates: 14g

Protein 2g

Matcha Coconut Smoothie

Serving: 2

Prep Time: 5 minutes

Cook Time: Nil

Ingredients:

1 whole banana, cubed

1 cup frozen mango, chunked

2 kale leaves, torn

3 tablespoons white beans

2 tablespoons shredded coconut

½ teaspoon Matcha green tea powder

1 cup water

How To:

1. Add banana, kale, mango, white beans, Matcha powder and white beans to the blender.

2. Blend until you have a nice smoothie.

3. Serve and enjoy!

Nutrition (Per Serving)

Calories: 200

Fat: 10g

Carbohydrates: 14g

Protein 2g

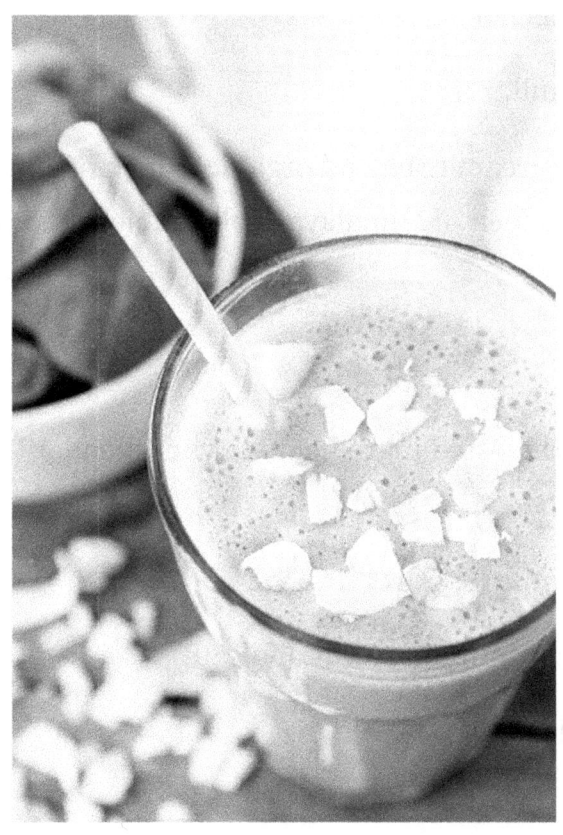

Ravishing Apple and Cucumber Glass

Serving: 2

Prep Time: 5 minutes

Ingredients:

1 green apple

2 cucumbers, peeled

1 cup almond milk

½ cup coconut cream (raw and organic) Pinch of cinnamon and nutmeg (each) Pinch of Himalayan salt 1 tablespoon coconut oil

How To:

1. Add all the listed ingredients to your blender (except oil, spices and salt).

2. Blend until smooth.

3. Mix in coconut oil, spices and salt.

4. Stir and enjoy!

Nutrition (Per Serving)

Calories: 200

Fat: 10

Carbohydrates: 14g

Protein 2g

Creative Winter Smoothie

Serving: 2

Prep Time: 5 minutes

Ingredients:

3 tomatoes, peeled

1 celery stalk

2 cloves garlic, peeled

1-inch ginger, peeled

1 cucumber, peeled

Juice of 1 lemon

1 cup alkaline water

Salt as needed

Pepper as needed

Pinch of turmeric

Olive oil/avocado oil

How To:

1. Add tomatoes, celery, garlic, cucumber and water to your blender.

2. Blend well until smooth.

3. Add lemon juice, salt and oil.

4. Stir.

5. Season with pepper and turmeric.

6. Stir.

7. Serve chilled and enjoy!

Nutrition (Per Serving)

Calories: 200

Fat: 10g

Carbohydrates: 14g

Protein 2g

The Hearty Garlic and Mushroom Crunch

Serving: 6

Prep Time: 10 minutes

Cooking Time: 8 hours

Ingredients:

¼ cup vegetable stock

2 tablespoons extra virgin olive oil

1 tablespoon Dijon mustard

1 teaspoon dried thyme

1 teaspoon sea salt

½ teaspoon dried rosemary

¼ teaspoon fresh ground black pepper

2 pounds cremini mushrooms, cleaned

6 garlic cloves, minced

¼ cup fresh parsley, chopped

How To:

1. Take a small bowl and whisk in vegetable stock, mustard, olive oil, salt, thyme, pepper and rosemary.

2. Add mushrooms, garlic and stock mix to your Slow Cooker.

3. Close lid and cook on LOW for 8 hours.

4. Open lid and stir in parsley.

5. Serve and enjoy!

Nutrition (Per Serving)

Calories: 92

Fat: 5g

Carbohydrates: 8g

Protein: 4g

Easy Pepper Jack Cauliflower

Serving: 6

Prep Time: 10 minutes

Cooking Time: 3 hours 35 minutes

Ingredients:

1 head cauliflower

¼ cup whipping cream 4 ounces cream cheese

½ teaspoon pepper

1 teaspoon salt

2 tablespoons butter

4 ounces pepper jack cheese

How To:

1. Grease slow cooker and add listed ingredients.
2. Stir and place lid, cook on LOW for 3 hours.
3. Remove lid and add cheese, stir.
4. Place lid and cook for 1 hour more.

5. Enjoy!

Nutrition (Per Serving)

Calories: 272

Fat: 21g

Carbohydrates: 5g

Protein: 10g

The Brussels Platter

Serving: 4

Prep Time: 15 minutes

Cooking Time: 4 hours

Ingredients:

1 pound Brussels sprouts, bottoms trimmed and cut

1 tablespoon olive oil

1 ½ tablespoons Dijon mustard

Salt and pepper to taste

½ teaspoon dried tarragon

How To:

1. Add Brussels sprouts, mustard, water, salt and pepper to your Slow Cooker

2. Add dried tarragon. 3. Stir well and cover.

3. Cook on LOW for 5 hours, making sure to keep cooking until the Brussels sprouts are tender.

4. Stir well and arrange.

5. Add Dijon over the Brussels sprouts.

6. Enjoy!

Nutrition (Per Serving)

Calories: 83

Fat: 4g

Carbohydrates: 11g

Protein: 4g

The Crazy Southern Salad

Serving: 2

Prep Time: 10 minutes

Cook Time: nil

Ingredients:

5 cups Romaine lettuce

½ cup sprouted black beans

1 cup cherry tomatoes, halved

1 avocado, diced

¼ cup almonds, chopped

½ cup of fresh cilantro

½ cup of Salsa Fresca

How To:

1. Take a large sized bowl and add lettuce, tomatoes, beans, almonds, cilantro, avocado, Salsa Fresco
2. Toss everything well and mix them

3. Divide the salad into serving bowls and serve!

4. Enjoy!

Nutrition (Per Serving)

Calories: 211

Fat: 16g

Carbohydrates: 6g

Protein: 10g

Kale and Carrot with Tahini Dressing

Serving: 1

Prep Time: 15 minutes

Cook Time: nil

Ingredients:

Handful of kale

1 tablespoon tahnini

½ head lettuce

Pinch of garlic powder

1 tablespoon olive oil

Juice of ½ lime

1 carrot, grated

How To:

1. Add kale and roughly chopped lettuce to a bowl.
2. Add grated carrots to the greens and mix.

3. Take a small bowl and add the remaining ingredients, mix well.

4. Pour dressing on top of greens and toss.

5. Enjoy!

Nutrition (Per Serving)

Calories: 249

Fat: 11g

Carbohydrates: 35g

Protein: 10g

Crispy Kale

Serving: 4

Prep Time: 10 minutes

Cook Time: 25 minutes

Ingredients:

3 cups kale, stemmed and thoroughly washed, torn in 2-inch pieces

1 tablespoon extra-virgin olive oil

½ teaspoon chili powder

¼ teaspoon sea salt

How To:

1. Prepare your oven by pre-heating to 300 degrees F.

2. Line 2 baking sheets with parchment paper and keep them on the side.

3. Dry kale and transfer to a large bowl.

4. Add olive oil and toss, making sure to cover the leaves well.

5. Season kale with salt, chili powder and toss.

6. Divide kale between baking sheets and spread into single layer.

7. Bake for 25 minutes until crispy.

8. Let them cool for 5 minutes, serve.

9. Enjoy!

Nutrition (Per Serving)

Calories: 56

Fat: 4g

Carbohydrates: 5g

Protein: 2g

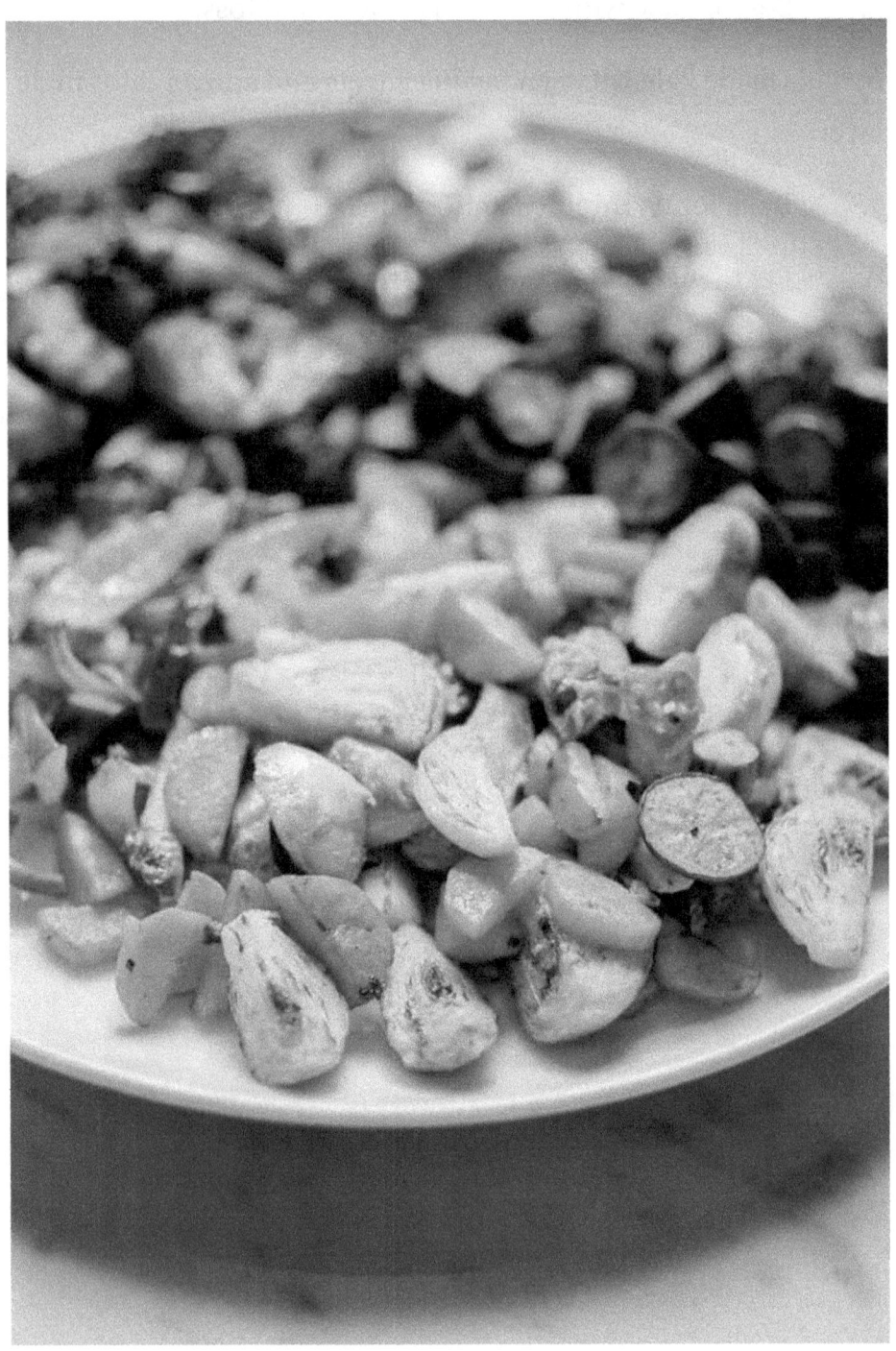

www.ingramcontent.com/pod-product-compliance
Lightning Source LLC
Chambersburg PA
CBHW071112030426
42336CB00013BA/2053